Mamadou Moustapha THIOUB
Sara NDIAYE

Referral and counter-referral in obstetric emergencies

Mamadou Moustapha THIOUB
Sara NDIAYE

Referral and counter-referral in obstetric emergencies

Obstetric referral in a context of isolation and excess maternal mortality in Kédougou, Senegal

ScienciaScripts

Imprint
Any brand names and product names mentioned in this book are subject to trademark, brand or patent protection and are trademarks or registered trademarks of their respective holders. The use of brand names, product names, common names, trade names, product descriptions etc. even without a particular marking in this work is in no way to be construed to mean that such names may be regarded as unrestricted in respect of trademark and brand protection legislation and could thus be used by anyone.

Cover image: www.ingimage.com

This book is a translation from the original published under ISBN 978-620-6-73234-1.

Publisher:
Sciencia Scripts
is a trademark of
Dodo Books Indian Ocean Ltd. and OmniScriptum S.R.L publishing group

120 High Road, East Finchley, London, N2 9ED, United Kingdom
Str. Armeneasca 28/1, office 1, Chisinau MD-2012, Republic of Moldova, Europe
Managing Directors: Ieva Konstantinova, Victoria Ursu
info@omniscriptum.com

Printed at: see last page
ISBN: 978-620-2-76036-2

SUMMARY

As part of the drive to improve primary healthcare, a referral and counter-referral system has been set up in Senegal to meet the needs of the population in terms of the quality of care provided.

The aim of this study is to describe the constraints linked to the smooth running of the referral and counter-referral system for obstetric emergencies at the Maternity Hospital of the Kédougou Health Centre.

This is a retrospective qualitative study to describe the qualitative aspects of the referral and counter-referral system in the Kédougou health district through individual interviews with qualified providers and the administration of a questionnaire to pregnant, labouring and post-partum women evacuated to the Maternity Unit of the Kédougou Health Centre in 2019.

The results showed that the referral and counter-referral system faces several constraints in the Kédougou health district. Delivery haemorrhage is the main obstetric emergency, accounting for 67% of referrals.

The telephone is the most frequently used means of informing the referral structure. 61% of patients referred are not accompanied by a qualified provider.

76% of the health workers surveyed considered the conditions for referring obstetric emergencies to be "very difficult", for various reasons. None of the facilities had a medical ambulance and 28% of health facilities did not have referral and counter-referral bulletins at the time of the survey.

The results of this study also showed a weakness in the monitoring and documentation of the reference and counter-reference system, with only 29% of providers completing the management tools in full.

These constraints described by providers and patients highlight the dysfunction of the referral and counter-referral system in the Kédougou health district.

The poor performance of the reference and counter-reference system is linked to weak monitoring and documentation.

Key words: Constraints; System; Reference-Counter-Reference; Obstetric emergencies.

TABLE OF CONTENTS

INTRODUCTION

Senegal's health policy is based on the Constitution, article 17 of which states that: "The State and public authorities have a duty to ensure the physical and moral health of the family and, in particular, of disabled and elderly people. The State guarantees families in general and those living in rural areas in particular access to health services and well-being [...] (Constitution of Senegal 2001)". Health is therefore a right guaranteed by the Senegalese Constitution, and to achieve this, the State of Senegal has set up a number of health plans, programmes and projects to give the entire population equitable access to health services. As part of the drive to improve primary healthcare, a referral and counter-referral system has been set up in Senegal to meet the needs of the population in terms of quality of care.

"Referral is the orientation and/or transfer of the patient to a higher level of the pyramid, accompanied by information on the patient's examination and/or the intervention carried out, for more appropriate care. As for counter-referral, this is the reorientation and/or return of the patient to the lower level of the health pyramid, accompanied by information on the patient's examination, the intervention carried out and the advice for correct follow-up", according to Senegal's national manual of strategies on referral and counter-referral. Following the Alma Ata conference (1978), the government of Senegal committed itself to achieving the Millennium Development Goals by, among other things, putting in place a good reference and counter-reference system. According to the national referral and counter-referral manual, "several evaluations of the performance of health structures have revealed shortcomings in the supply and demand for health services, including the absence of a formal framework and indicators for monitoring referral and counter-referral.

The criteria for a good reference and counter-reference system are as follows, according to Senegal's national manual of reference and counter-reference strategies:

• The existence of a national health map with the various health structures complementing each other to provide better care for referred cases;
• Good organisation of work in health facilities, with well-trained staff who are familiar with treatment protocols;
• Adequate means of transport (medical ambulance);
• Collaboration and coordination between all health structures through a good information ;
• Regular formative supervision.

Any patient in need of special care should be referred in the best possible conditions, and counter-referred at the end of their hospital stay to ensure proper follow-up. However, it has been observed that the application of referral and counter-referral is a real problem at all levels of the Senegalese health pyramid.

The aim of this study is to describe the constraints linked to the smooth running of the referral and counter-referral system for obstetric emergencies at the Maternity Hospital of the Kédougou Health Centre from January to December 2019.
More specifically, this involved :

• To carry out a situational analysis of referral and counter-referral of obstetric emergencies at the Maternity Unit of the Kédougou Health Centre.

• Describe the conditions referral and counter-referral of obstetric emergencies from the providers' point of view.

• To explain the conditions for referral and counter-referral of obstetric emergencies from the point of view of those referred.

The Maternity Ward at the Kédougou Health Centre was the only referral facility in the region in 2019. It played the role of a regional hospital centre, receiving all obstetric emergencies referred by other health facilities. Today, we can see that the people of Kédougou, without this being backed up by a qualitative survey, are complaining about difficulties in accessing hospital care and even about the quality of services offered at the Maternity Ward of the Kédougou Health Centre. We therefore proposed to carry out a study on the constraints linked to the smooth running of the referral and counter-referral in order to understand these constraints. As part of this study, we propose to describe the constraints linked to the smooth running of the referral and counter-referral system for obstetric emergencies at the Maternity Hospital of the Kédougou Health Centre in 2019.
In order to describe these constraints, we first described the problem of the reference and counter-reference system in two aspects: the reference versus counter-reference in question and the emergencies in the reference versus counter-reference. After announcing the issue and the research hypothesis, the literature review was discussed. In this second chapter, we began with a review of retrospective descriptive studies, followed by a conceptual clarification before presenting our research methodology, which forms the third chapter of this dissertation.

We then analysed and interpreted the data. These different aspects were studied:

• Providers' views on the reference and counter-reference system.

• The point of view of referrers on the reference and counter-reference system.

• The three delays in the reference and counter-reference system.

• Weaknesses in the monitoring and documentation of the reference and counter-reference system.

• Providers' suggestions improving the referral and counter-referral system reference.

Once the data had been analysed and interpreted, the practical aspects were described in Chapter 6 before drawing the general conclusion of the study.

CHAPTER 1

PROBLEMATIC

1.1. REFERENCE AND COUNTER-REFERENCE

Maternal mortality remains a global concern. The death of a woman during the gravid-puerperal period is a dreaded event for society, a distressing ordeal that results in large number of orphans, loss of income, and contributes to the impoverishment of families and society. Children often die in infancy, and for those who survive, their education is seriously compromised (Ngom, N. F. 2016).

Maternal mortality, which has become rare in developed countries, is a public health problem in developing countries where the reference and counter-reference system is unsatisfactory (Diallo, A. et al. 2019).

In 2015, around 10.7 million maternal deaths were recorded worldwide between 1999 and 2015. 99% of these deaths occurred in developing countries, two-thirds of them in sub-Saharan Africa, according to a report by the World Health Organisation. (WHO 2015).

In operational terms, there are many factors limiting the performance of the reference and counter-reference system.

Counter-referral" seems to be poorly rooted in the professional culture of providers and almost meaningless for patients [...]. [Most of the patients referred to the next level do not return to their original facility after their operation. Some of the patients interviewed ignore the referral altogether, or even consider it inappropriate to return to the facility that referred them because they have recovered. This situation is the result of a lack of communication between healthcare providers and patients" (VANCUTSEM, I. 2011).

A qualitative study carried out in Mali on the problems of the referral and counter-referral system for obstetric emergencies and the involvement of communities in the district of Bamako in 2015 revealed "shortcomings, particularly in the conditions under which patients are transferred. Furthermore, the lack of community involvement is a major handicap to the proper functioning of the referral/counter-referral system". (Théra, T. et al. 2015). Research conducted at Parakou University Hospital in Benin showed that only 2.2% of patients received medical transport. The other means of transport were: public transport cars (78.9%), motorbikes (9.9%) and fire brigade vehicles (9%) (Tchaou, B. A., 2015). At the national workshop on referral versus counter-referral held in Diourbel under the auspices of the Senegalese Ministry of Health, the main problems identified in the referral and counter-referral system in Senegal were as follows:

6

• Insufficient collaboration between PHE and the medical region ;

• Inadequate development of staff knowledge and skills ;

• Delay in taking a decision on the reference at Community level ;

• Lack of financial support for referred patients;

• Inadequate and irregular monitoring/evaluation of the benchmark/counter-benchmark;

• Absence or break of bulletins from reference/counter reference and register evacuations.

1.2. EMERGENCIES IN REFERENCE AND COUNTER REFERENCE REFERENCE

A study on referral and counter-referral of obstetric emergencies carried out in Senegal showed that "evacuation was carried out using an ambulance only in 69% of cases and this was accompanied by an unqualified provider in 92.7% of cases. The lack of resources on the part of both the community and the healthcare staff seems to be at the heart of all the problems" (Thiam, O. 2014) Some providers believe that the problems of the referral and counter-referral system are exacerbated "insufficient coordination of referral and counter-referral activities". Indeed, "the monitoring and evaluation of the referral and counter-referral system is never on the agenda at health facility coordination meetings". An evaluation of the obstetric referral and counter-referral system in Guinea from [1]August 2017 to 31 January 2018 revealed that "out of 560 referrals received in the department, the referral protocol was never complied with in full". Also according to this evaluation, "33% of these referrals were not justified and more than 63% of the reasons for referral did not agree with the definitive diagnosis retained at the referral Maternity Hospital" (Théra, T. et al. 2015). According to a study carried out on the problems of the referral and counter-referral system for obstetric emergencies and the involvement of communities in the district of Bamako, "50.6% of patients are evacuated by ambulance and 15.4% of these patients are accompanied by health staff at the time of referral. This unassisted transport of women evacuees, who were sometimes in a state of shock, contributed to darkening their vital prognosis." (Diallo, A. et al. 2019). A study carried out at the Thiès regional hospital centre showed that the proportion of women at risk of maternal death was 78% among evacuated women. In addition, four factors (late arrival, absence or slowness of the provider, late transfer to the appropriate level of care, and late correct diagnosis) were studied and all contributed to 42.2% of maternal deaths (THIAM, M. 2017)."Maternal and perinatal mortality is a major public health problem in developing countries." (Diallo, A. et al. 2019). In 2017, perinatal mortality was 250 per

100,000 live births in Kédougou region, compared with a national average of 236 per 100,000 live births (PNDSS 2019-2028 page 15). This rate, which is higher than the national average, highlights the difficulties involved in dealing with obstetric emergencies, because if the referral and counter-referral for obstetric emergencies had been efficient, some of these deaths could have been avoided. In 2019, according to the report on curative activities at the Salémata Health Centre, 24 patients were evacuated to the Maternity Unit at the Kédougou Health Centre, including 7 for severe anaemia and 7 for eclampsia. of these 24 referrals received a counter-referral from the Maternity Unit at the Kédougou Health Centre, and yet all of these referrals were evacuated by ambulance with a referral/counter-referral form. The absence of a counter-referral does not contribute to the complete management of the patients evacuated, as the latter, suffering from severe anaemia, eclampsia, the threat of premature abortion or dystocic labour, need to be followed up at the facility that referred them to enable them to avoid relapses. In Kédougou, the counter-reference is very problematic. It is exceptional to receive a counter-referral. It is up to the higher level to send the counter-referral, as this is of vital importance in patient follow-up. However, the Ministry of Health has drawn up a reference/counter-reference document to facilitate the systematisation of counter-referrals, but it has been observed that most providers do not carry out this task. Sometimes the health worker is obliged to call on the telephone to obtain further information about the counter-referral. The counter-referral contributes to the ongoing training of the referring healthcare workers. By not receiving a counter-reference, they miss out on an opportunity to continue their training.

1.3. QUESTION FOR RESEARCH

What are the constraints on the smooth running of the referral and counter-referral system for obstetric emergencies at the Maternity Unit of the Kédougou Health Centre?

1.4. RESEARCH HYPOTHESIS

The poor performance of the reference and counter-reference system is linked to the weakness of the monitoring and documentation of the reference and counter-reference.

Researchers have always been interested in the reference system as a way of finding answers to this problem. The literature review enabled us to gain a better understanding of the aspects linked to the reference and counter-reference system, but also to consult and exploit the necessary documents relating to the theme of this study, thus enabling us to make an inventory of the scientific work already carried out in relation to the reference and counter-reference . In fact, we looked through a large number of documents relating to our study topic. During this documentary research, we visited several research sites, which enabled us to see that the issue of the reference and counter-reference system had been the subject of several studies. The resulting analysis led us to review some of the literature in this field. Already in 2014, a prospective study on the difficulties encountered by parturients evacuated to a rural area in Senegal showed that, despite limited resources, it is possible to manage and reduce the morbidity and mortality of evacuated patients if an obstetric UAS system in rural areas is set up (Thiam, O. 2014).

The evaluation of the referral/evacuation system for obstetric emergencies in Commune IV of the Bamako district in Mali described, among other things, the organisation and operation of the referral/evacuation system in the Commune IV health district in Bamako. According to the study, continuous improvement of the referral/evacuation system has led to a reduction in the maternal death rate. However, the sustainability of the system is threatened by the non-payment of contributions by certain players in the system (N'golo, F. 2018). Another study on the problems of the referral/evacuation system for obstetric emergencies at the referral health centre in Commune VI, Bamako, reveals that various parameters influence the prognosis of evacuees: distance travelled, evacuation conditions, economic conditions, age, parity, reason for evacuation. Still according to the results of his studies, the qualification of the agent who decides on evacuation is part of the aspects linked to the problem and this poses the problem of competence and the equipment at his disposal. In 724 cases, or 76.37% of those evacuated, the reason was not consistent with the diagnosis (Traore, D. 2010). In a study of the determinants of obstetric complications, the link between the occurrence of obstetric complications and the means of transport used and obstetric evacuation was highlighted. The aim of this study was to identify the factors associated with obstetric complications in parturients admitted to the two maternity units of Conakry University Hospital. The means of transport used at the time of referral had a significant impact on the occurrence of obstetric complications. The more adequate the means of transport, the more likely the referred patient was to avoid obstetric complications (Baldé et al. 2019).

An evaluation of the obstetric referral and counter-referral system at the Ignace Deen Maternity Hospital in Guinea showed that the referral and counter-referral process has several shortcomings both at the referring centre and at the Ignace Deen Maternity Hospital. These shortcomings worsen the maternal prognosis for women referred, as the referral protocol has never been fully complied with. All evacuees were found to have undergone at least one activity that was not carried out at all or not adequately, either during preparation by the referring centre or during transport from the emergency to the referral maternity unit. A third of the referrals made were not relevant insofar as in the referring facilities, the conditions were met to ensure on-site management of the cases. (Diallo et al. 2019).

A prospective study of the obstetric referral/evacuation system at the Banamba referral health centre showed that setting up a referral/evacuation system combined with free Caesarean sections reduced the rate of maternal and foetal deaths. However, there are still problems with the referral/evacuation system:

• Non-payment of contributions by local authorities;

• Delayed evacuation: poor road conditions; initial reluctance on the parturient's or her parents' part;

• Communication: disrupted telephone networks (Touré, S. 2019).

The results of the work on the problems of the reference and counter-reference system showed that evacuation and unfavourable socio-economic conditions are the main problems listed in the problems of the reference and counter-reference system (Traoré, A. T. 2014).

Research at the Cotonou University Clinic of Gynaecology and Obstetrics (CUGO) in 2015 led to a better understanding of the reasons for opting out of obstetric referral. The problem of not seeking emergency obstetric care at the CUGO is based on social, organisational, geographical, economic and cultural factors. The poor quality of information held by women on the reasons for referral, the fear of caesarean section perceived as obvious and the difficult relations with the health staff contribute to referral avoidance. In addition, rumours circulating about the reception, delays in treatment and conditions of hospitalisation at the CUGO are aspects to be taken into account. Finally, the distance from which the referral originates is a determining factor in the acceptance of the referral by women and their families (Houngnihin, R. A., & Sossou, A. J. (2017).

An evaluation of the referral/evacuation system focusing on obstetric emergencies from 2015 to 2018 in the Yelimané health district showed that gesity and parity play an important role in the cause of evacuations. The 36.21% of evacuees were in their first pregnancy, while 11.48% were in their 6th or more. Nulliparous women were the most evacuated, at 32.58% (Dembélé, H. 2020). A descriptive cross-sectional study carried out in the Democratic Republic of Congo showed that the referral system was dysfunctional, with referrals being made almost without reference notes, and hospitals not cross-referring patients (Kafuku, M. 2016).

CHAPTER 3

CONCEPTUAL FRAMEWORK

The literature suggests a conceptual clarification of the following terms: system, reference, counter-reference, health pyramid, reference/counter-reference system, evacuation and feedback.

A. **SYSTEM:** It is defined as the people, institutions and resources, brought together by established policies, to improve the health of the population they serve [...] (WHO, 2017). Senegal's healthcare system is made up of 03 levels:

❖ The central level, which includes the Minister's Office, the General Secretariat, the Directorates-General, the National Directorates and the central services.

National Social Reinsertion Centres and level 3 Public Health Establishments;

❖ The strategic intermediary level, which brings together the Medical Regions, the Brigades Régionales de l'Hygiène (BRH), Services Régionaux de l'Action

Social Security (SRAS) and level 2 Public Health Establishments;

❖ The operational peripheral level with the Health Districts, the Hygiene Sub-Brigades, Departmental Social Action Departments, the Health and Social Services Departments, etc. Centres de Promotion et de Réinsertion Sociale (CPRS) and level 1 Public Health Establishments.

The provision of healthcare follows the architecture of the health pyramid. At the top, the PHCs constitute the last level of reference, followed by health centres at the intermediate level and health posts at the peripheral level. This system is supplemented by the private sector, traditional medicine and, at community level, by health centres.

There are forty (40) PHEs, 36 of them hospital-based and 04 non-hospital-based. They are grouped into three levels.

Senegal is divided into 77 health districts comprising 102 health ; 1,415 health posts including 2,676 health huts in 2018 (PNDSS 2018_2029).

The WHO, in its publication entitled "Recommendations for clinical practice in emergency obstetric and neonatal care in Africa: a provider's guide third edition (2018) offers us the following definitions of concepts:

B. **REFERRAL:** this is the mechanism by which a maternity unit refers a patient who is beyond its competence to a more specialised and better-equipped facility (usually a hospital)

for appropriate care.

C. **COUNTER REFERRAL**: this is the mechanism by which a more specialised and better-equipped facility refers a patient to the maternity unit that referred her, to ensure continuity of care and post-hospital follow-up.

D. **THE SYSTEM FROM REFERENCE/COUNTER REFERENCE** :is all the measures taken to ensure the two-way flow (to and fro) of patients between two care structures with different levels of competence, in order to provide patients with the care they need, in the right place and at the right time.

E. **EVACUATION**: by convention, this term is used to designate a referral made in an emergency situation. This is the case for emergency obstetric and neonatal care (EmONC).

F. **RETRO INFORMATION OR "FEED-BACK"**: is the response given by the referral facility to the health facility which referred the patient. It includes information on the patient's reception, the diagnosis made, the care administered and the prescriptions for continuing treatment.

The African Society of Obstetrics and Gynaecology (SAGO) adopted the following definitions at its biannual conference in Dakar in 1998:

❖ Operational definition Referral/evacuation: This is the mechanism by which a

A peripheral health facility refers a case that is beyond its remit to a better-equipped facility. The referral/evacuation process involves the following stages: - Preparation of the emergency by the referring centre (using the referral form, informing the parents, inserting a venous line) - Transport of the patient (medical vehicle, accompanied by an agent and medical care during transport) - Reception of the patient at the referring maternity hospital.

❖ Counter-referral: This is the process put in place to ensure feedback.

from a referral facility which has received a patient for more specific care to the facility which referred the patient. The feedback form should describe: the origin of the transfer, the diagnosis made, the care received and the course of treatment, and recommendations regarding any shortcomings identified during care at the peripheral facility (Boré, B. (2021).

G. HEALTH PYRAMID

Senegal's healthcare system is pyramid-shaped, with the community level at the base and the level 3 PHEs at the top of the pyramid, which are the last level in the CRRS. The community level is the first stage in the CRRCS. It is made up exclusively of community staff (ACs, ACPPs) with the following health structures: community sites and health huts. The first level of reference for community structures is the health post. This is the second rung of Senegal's health pyramid, and in addition to community staff, it is staffed by EDPs and FHTs who refer their patients to the health centre. If no services are available at the health centre, the patient must be referred to a level 1 PHE, which in turn refers to a level 2 PHE if no care is available for the referred patient. PHE2s, in turn, refer to level 3 PHEs if the care required by the patient's condition is not available at PHE2 level.

The conceptual framework of Senegal's referral and counter-referral system is based on the pyramid style to facilitate patient referral and counter-referral (see Appendix 4).

CHAPTER 4

METHODOLOGY

4.1. STUDY SETTING: THE KEDOUGOU HEALTH CENTRE

Created in 1962, the Kédougou Health Centre is the administrative centre of the Kédougou health district. It is located in the Gomba district, on Route Nationale 7. It is bordered to the north by the RN7, to the east by the kindergarten, to the west by the Kédougou power station and to the south by the Catholic mission. It has a population of 25,476 and serves as a referral centre for the Saraya and Salémata districts. Because of its geographical position, it receives patients from neighbouring countries (Republic of Guinea Conakry and Mali).

In operation since 1962, the Maternity Ward of the Health Centre consists of :

• A consultation and ultrasound room for the gynaecologist;

• A 15-bed hospital ;

• A recovery room / caesarean section with 5 beds;

• A humanised delivery with 01 bed;

• An emergency room with 05 beds;

• Three examination cubicles;

• One on-call room with 01 bed;

• The midwife's office;

• An ultrasound ;

• A room.

❖ **HUMAN RESOURCES**

The Maternity Unit is staffed by a gynaecologist and obstetrician, 11 midwives, including 6 civil servants (head midwife, coordinator and four other midwives) and 5 community midwives, 11 matrons, including 7 Bajenu Gox and 4 relays.

❖ **ORGANISATION AND OPERATION OF THE MATERNITY**

Maternity services are permanent, with a team of midwives call every 12 hours, assisted by matrons under the supervision of the head of department. The Maternity Ward is organised as follows

• ANC, ONC, FP activities, deliveries and hospitalisations

• Ultrasound scans

• Prevention and health promotion activities.

The department is run by an obstetrician-gynaecologist. The MSF is responsible for organising and coordinating activities, the other midwives are responsible for providing care and the matrons, some of whom are also Bajenu Gox or relays, are responsible for awareness-raising activities.

An analysis of the situation at the Maternity Ward of the Kédougou Health Centre revealed :

• Lack medical ambulances used exclusively for evacuating

obstetric emergencies.

• Only one gynaecologist and 11 state midwives for 6,116 women of reproductive age, whereas the World Health Organisation recommends one gynaecologist for every 10,000 inhabitants and one midwife for every 3,000 inhabitants.

• Lack of an operational referral system between different levels of care

(primary, secondary and tertiary).

• Only 50% of midwives trained in EmONC (basic emergency obstetric and neonatal care)

• No guidance or training for community players on referral and counter-referral.

4.2. POPULATION OF STUDY

The study population consisted of :

• The Chief Medical Officer of the Kédougou health district.

• The gynaecologist at the Maternity Unit of the Kédougou Health Centre.

• The midwives at the Maternity Ward of the Kédougou Health Centre.

• Head nurses and midwives from health posts in the Kédougou health district.

• All pregnant women in labour or post-partum who are evacuated to the Maternity Ward of the Kédougou Health Centre in 2019.

4.3. SAMPLING

To analyse the constraints linked to the smooth running of the referral and counter-referral system for obstetric emergencies at the Maternity Hospital of the Kédougou Health Centre, we adopted a qualitative methodology. In order to obtain an overall view of the constraints linked to the smooth running of the referral and counter-referral system, we used the principle of diversification as described by Alvaro Pires in his book entitled "Échantillonnage et qualitative research: a theoretical and methodological essay. Qualitative research. Epistemological and methodological issues", which we followed.

We inventoried all the stakeholder profiles involved. This enabled us to identify, from the outset of our exploration :

- Patients: identified on the basis of reference registers from the health posts. A total of 51 women were interviewed.
- The Chief Medical Officer at the Kédougou health centre: he was on duty at the facility throughout the 2019 reference year.
- The gynaecologist at the Kédougou health centre: he was on duty at the facility throughout the reference year.
- Midwives at health posts and the Kédougou health centre: they were identified from the directory of health post staff. There were 22 midwives interviewed, all in service during the reference year.
- KPIs: These were identified from the health post staff directory. A total of 12 were interviewed, all in service during the reference year.

Moreover, dictated by the principle of saturation described by Alvaro Pires, we surveyed 51 patients, and stopped collecting data within this category. Redundancy of information in the respondents' answers was sufficient as a criterion.

Given the limited number of qualified personnel in the Kédougou health district, they were all selected in full. However, due to the unavailability of some during the data collection period for this study, not all qualified providers in the Kédougou health district could be surveyed.

4.4. ETHICAL CONSIDERATIONS

This study was authorised by the approval committee of the Gaston Berger University of Saint Louis. Data collection also received the agreement of the Chief Medical Officer of the Kédougou health district. The participants in this study were informed before the start of the interviews of the confidentiality and anonymity of their responses, and each gave verbal consent. We are not aware of any conflicts of interest.

4.5. TECHNIQUES AND TOOLS FOR COLLECTION

To check whether the poor performance of the reference and counter-reference system is linked to the weakness of the monitoring and documentation of the reference and counter-reference, we used the following data collection protocol:

• Exploring documents (evacuation registers/books, referral/counter-referral forms, reports entered into the DHIS2) from the health posts and health centre in the Kédougou health district.

• The administration of a questionnaire to pregnant, labouring and post-partum women evacuated to the Maternity Unit of the Kédougou Health Centre in 2019.

• The use of an interview guide among qualified providers in the Kédougou health district.

Data collection was based on individual interviews using a patient questionnaire. As most were illiterate, the questions were asked orally and the answers recorded instantly. As for the providers who took part in this study, data was collected remotely by administering a written questionnaire. Once the data had been collected, Excel 2016 was used to analyse and interpret it.

CHAPTER 5

RESULTS

5.1. THE VIEWPOINT OF SERVICE PROVIDERS

The referral and counter-referral system is one of the issues discussed by most of the health workers in Kédougou, who are experiencing numerous difficulties in evacuating or receiving a counter-referral.

5.1.1. MAIN OBSTETRICAL EMERGENCIES REFERRED BY SERVICE POINTS IN THE KÉDOUGOU HEALTH DISTRICT

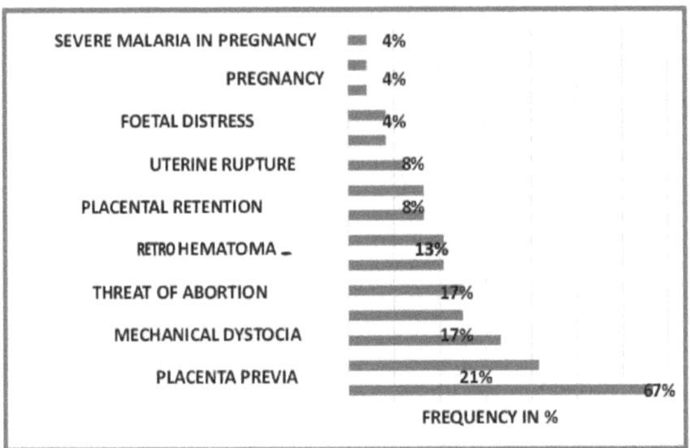

Figure 1: Main obstetric emergencies referred in the Kédougou health district in 2019.

According to the results of this study, delivery haemorrhage is the main obstetric emergency referred in the Kédougou health district (67% of referrals). Given the complications that can arise from a delivery haemorrhage, the referral and counter-referral system should not suffer from any malfunction. It should be operational and efficient at all levels, so that referrals can be made without delay and under the best possible conditions in the Kédougou health district.

5.1.2. INFORMATION RESOURCES FOR THE HOST STRUCTURE

The telephone is the most frequently used means of informing the host facility of the referral decision. All the providers take care to inform the reception centre by telephone before the patient leaves. The referral and counter-referral system standards require that referrals be made with a duly completed referral and counter-referral form and that the referred patient be accompanied by a qualified provider. However, the results of this study show that only 29%

of referred patients are accompanied by a qualified provider. Instead of a qualified provider, a matron accompanies the patient. In addition, 38% of healthcare facilities do not have reference and counter-reference forms. Instead, a handwritten note is drawn up to replace the reference and counter-reference form.

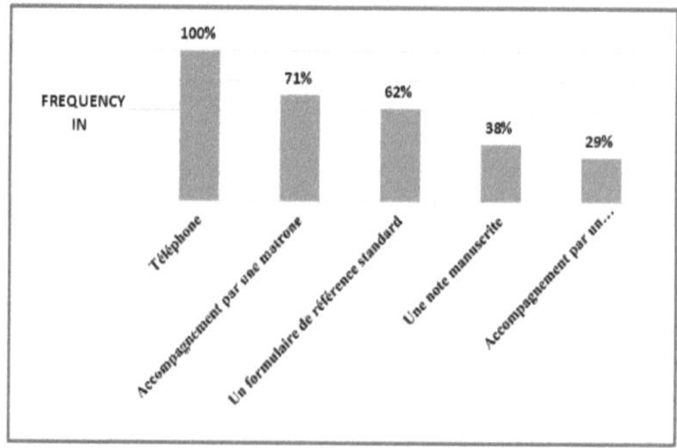

Figure 2: Information resources at the reception

5.1.3. PREPARATION OF EVACUATION

The level of preparation of the reference is positively assessed by all of the providers who took part in this study. All of the providers said that they use the algorithms in the MSAS policies, protocols and standards for the management of obstetric emergencies and that they decide on referral by ensuring that :

• The patient is well stabilised prior to transport (emergency medication available).

• The family has received full information about the referral arrangements.

• Transport is carried out quickly, safely and promptly.

• The host organisation is informed of the decision to refer before the the patient's departure.

5.1.4. THE AVAILABILITY OF REFERENCE AND COUNTER-REFERENCE SYSTEM MANAGEMENT TOOLS

All the management tools for the reference and counter-reference system provided by the Senegalese Ministry of Health and Social Action are not available in all the health facilities in the Kédougou health district. According to this study, 38% of facilities do not have two-part reference/counter-reference bulletins. A handwritten note is used instead of a two-part referral/counter-referral form, and only 29% of facilities have an evacuation register/book.

The other facilities that do not have one do not record the reference information on any tool.

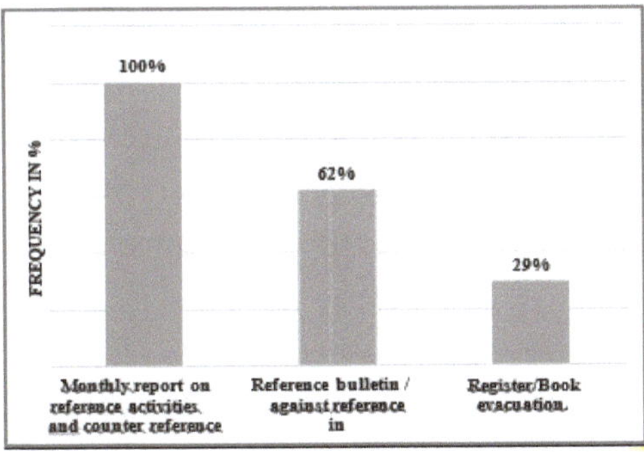

Figure 3: Availability of management tools

5.1.5. THE COUNTER REFERENCE

During this study, all providers stated that they had never been informed that a patient had been counter-referred. Admittedly, all of the providers found the counter-referral useful and felt that it contributed to the correct management of the patient. However, the observation made during this study is that the referral structures do not at all inform the referring structure that the patient has been counter-referred.

5.1.6. REFERENCE CONDITIONS FOR EMERGENCIES OBSTETRICAL EMERGENCIES

Assessments of referral conditions for obstetric emergencies in the Kédougou health district differ from one provider to another. None of the providers gave a positive assessment of referral conditions. 76% of the health workers surveyed judged the conditions for referral of obstetric emergencies to be "very difficult". The difficulties are related to the lack of passable roads. The majority of health posts are in rural areas, and with the very uneven terrain of the Kédougou region, evacuating a pregnant or post-partum woman in the best possible conditions is becoming a headache providers in the Kédougou health district. In addition, 3% of providers feel that the "system is poorly organised" because, according to them, there is no system of regulation between the health posts and the Maternity Ward of the Kédougou Health Centre. Another negative assessment of referral conditions is "the lack of qualified human resources" to accompany patients during evacuation. According to the results of this study, 71% of referrals are not accompanied by qualified staff. Given the complications that

21

can arise from obstetric emergencies, it is imperative to refer patients with qualified staff. However, given the lack of qualified staff in the Kédougou health district, some providers are obliged to have the patient accompanied by a matron, who is not sufficiently equipped to deal with any complications.In Kédougou, the cost of referral is borne by the patients, which is contrary to the recommendation of the health authorities. However, this situation is due to "a lack of financial resources on the part of the Health Development Committees", according to the providers.

"The lack of a medical ambulance is one of the reasons why providers are not satisfied with the conditions of the referral. None of the facilities in the Kédougou health district has a medical ambulance. Instead of a medical ambulance, simple ambulances are used for evacuations, and these do not guarantee compliance with patient transport standards and procedures.

5.2. THE POINT OF VIEW OF REFEREES

5.2.1. THE TIME ARRIVAL IN THE DEPARTMENT AND DECISION TO EVACUATE THE PATIENT

In the course of our study, 51 pregnant, labouring or postpartum women who were evacuated to the Maternity Unit of the Kédougou Health Centre in 2019 were the subject of data collection using a questionnaire. Of the 51 people surveyed, 53% were satisfied with the time between arrival on the ward and the decision to evacuate. However, 20% of patients were dissatisfied and 27% were not very satisfied. Of the reasons for dissatisfaction, 54% felt that the waiting time between their arrival and the decision to discharge them was too long. A further 20% were dissatisfied or not very satisfied because of the absence of a midwife at the health centre.

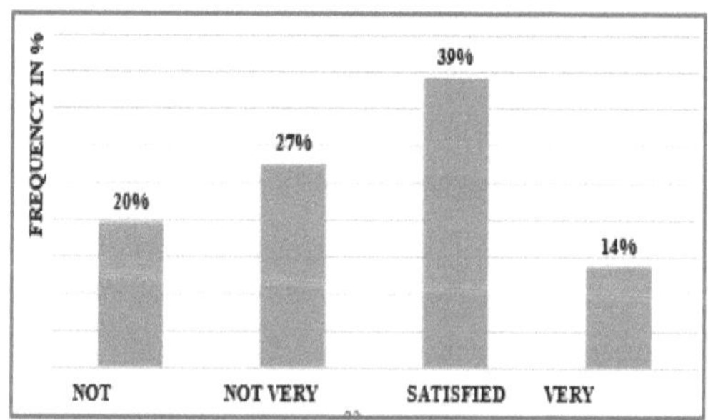

Graph 4: Level of satisfaction with the time taken to make the decision to evacuate patients

5.2.2. ASSESSMENT OF THE QUALITY OF EMERGENCY CARE OBSTETRICS

The quality emergency obstetric care at the Maternity Unit of the Kédougou Health Centre is assessed in different ways. The majority of patients (53%) were satisfied, while 47% were dissatisfied. For most patients (33%), the reason for dissatisfaction was the length of time it took from their arrival at the facility to their treatment. In addition, 21% of patients are dissatisfied because of the lack of a reception and referral service at the Maternity Ward of the Kédougou Health Centre.

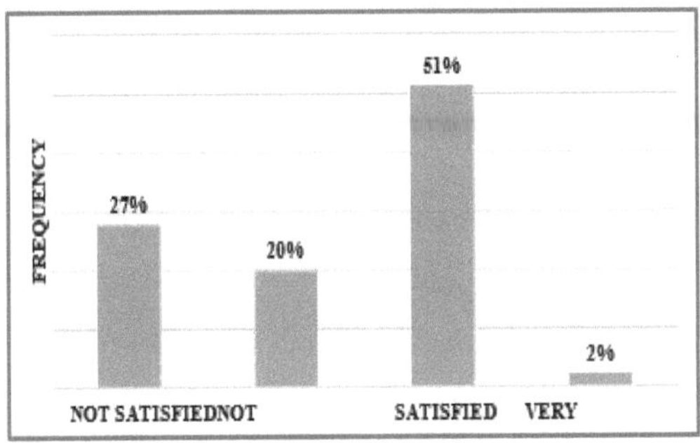

Graph 5: Level of satisfaction with the quality of emergency obstetric care.

5.2.3. ASSESSMENT OF REFERRAL CONDITIONS FOR OBSTETRIC EMERGENCIES

Of the 51 patients surveyed, 41% were satisfied with the referral conditions and 2% were very satisfied. However, 29% were not at all satisfied and 28% were not very satisfied. The reasons for dissatisfaction with the conditions of the obstetric emergency referral were mainly (52%) related to the cost of the referral borne by the patient. The other reason for dissatisfaction with referral conditions was the absence of an ambulance. 57% of patients were dissatisfied or not very satisfied because of the lack of a medical ambulance in their health facility. In 2019, during the period of our survey, no facility had a medical ambulance.

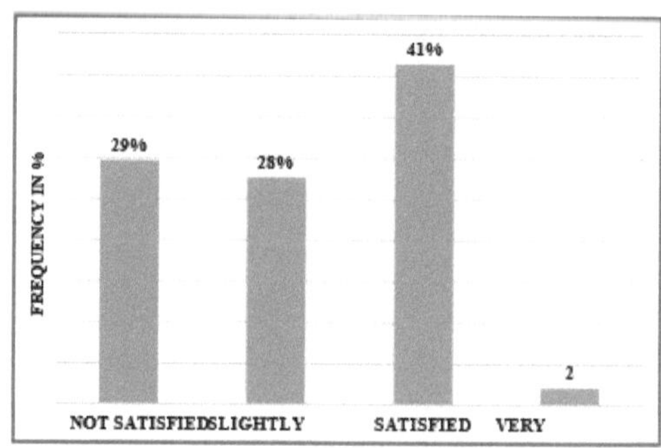

Graph 6: Level appreciation of obstetric emergency referral conditions.

5.3. THE DELAY IN TAKING A DECISION BY REFERENCE

In the reference and counter-reference system, there are three types of delay:

▪ **The first delay**: Recognising and taking the decision to look for care.

▪ **The second delay**: Transport to the care centre, delay on the way to an appropriate health facility.

▪ **The third delay**: the delay in receiving appropriate care at the referral health facility as soon as possible.

5.3.1. THE DELAY ATTRIBUTABLE TO MATERNITY CARE PROVIDERS AT THE KEDOUGOU HEALTH CENTRE

The third type of delay is attributable to health service providers. As the region's only referral facility for obstetric emergencies in 2019, the Maternity Ward of the Kédougou Health Centre had only one operating theatre to deal with all referred obstetric emergencies. Added to this is the lack of qualified human resources. The Maternity Unit at the Kédougou Health Centre had only one gynaecologist for the entire Kédougou region.

The high cost of emergency obstetric care is a determining factor in the third type of delay in the referral system in Kédougou. The results of this study showed that 43% of patients referred felt that their standard of living was low.

Another significant factor in the delay attributable to providers is the shortage of essential maternal health drugs. In discussions with practitioners, it is often noted that essential drugs for treating obstetric emergencies have run out. Although the Kédougou health centre has a blood bank, there is often a serious shortage of blood or blood derivatives. In fact, this study showed that 67% of obstetric emergencies referred to the Maternity Unit of the Kédougou Health Centre are linked to delivery haemorrhage, hence the increased need for blood products. However, blood donation is not part of the culture of the people of Kédougou. The low level of support for blood donation remains a major obstacle to the availability of blood products. In this study, 100% of the providers interviewed felt that there was a fairly long delay (more than 30 minutes) between the patient's arrival and the referral decision.

Furthermore, the patients with the highest success rate were those evacuated on time, and the maternal deaths recorded were very often linked to delays in the decision to refer.

5.3.2. DELAYS ATTRIBUTABLE TO PATIENTS

Recognition and the decision to seek care are the first delays, and this concerns the whole population. This delay is often linked to a lack of awareness of the danger signs on the part of the community, but poverty and low levels of education are also among the reasons for not seeking care. Analysis of the results of this study shows that 43% of the patients surveyed have a low standard of living. The high cost of treating obstetric emergencies means that some people prefer to self-medicate rather than go to the Kédougou health centre. The results of the Harmonised Survey of Household Living Conditions (EHCVM 2018/2019) in Senegal showed that in rural areas, self-medication is cited by 37.4% of the rural population as a reason for not using health facilities.

The level of education is also one of the determinants of delay attributable to patients. A number of surveys have shown that the less educated a person is, the less likely they are to use health services in case of need. There is a strong correlation between the level of education and the decision to use a health facility in case of need. In the Kédougou health district, the majority of the population lives in rural areas (82%) and 47% of the population has no schooling, according to the results of this study.

Socio-cultural aspects are among the factors identified as favouring the occurrence of the first delay. In rural areas (especially in the Kédougou health district), women are not autonomous in their decision-making. It is the mothers-in-law who decide whether or not to consult a health facility. As they are unaware of the danger signs of pregnancy, they are very late making decision to seek care in health facilities.

5.4. WEAKNESSES IN MONITORING AND DOCUMENTATION OF THE REFERENCE AND COUNTER-REFERENCE

During the course of this study on the constraints linked to the smooth running of the referral and counter-referral system for obstetric emergencies at the Maternity Unit of the Kédougou Health Centre in 2019, several weaknesses in the monitoring and documentation of referral and counter-referral were noted. A referral and counter-referral system cannot function properly without the availability of management tools. These tools enable all the information needed to facilitate reception at the referral structure to be recorded. They also make it possible to collect all the information needed to monitor and evaluate the referral and counter-referral system. In the Kédougou health district, all the health facilities had a monthly report on referral and counter-referral activities. This tool is part of the document known as the "global zone report" for service delivery points. However, the evacuation register/book was only present in 29% of health facilities. This enables a great deal of information to be collected on the patient, such as the reasons for referral, the conditions of evacuation, the time of arrival and the time of the decision to evacuate, the examinations or treatment administered to the patient, etc.In addition, the two-part referral and counter-referral form is only present in 62% of health facilities, whereas the latter, given its importance, should be present in all health facilities, even at community level. The MSAS has drawn up a document for this purpose, known as the "referral and counter-referral form", to record all the necessary information so that the receiving facility has all the information it needs to provide correct and rapid care for the referred patient. The second part of the referral and counter-referral form also plays a vital role at the time of the counter-referral, as it contains useful information about the patient to ensure proper follow-up at the referring facility.

5.5. EXHAUSTIVE COMPLETION OF ALL THE ITEMS IN THE REGISTER AND THE REFERENCE BULLETIN AND AGAINST REFERENCE

Even if the reference and counter-reference system management tools exist in the structure, they are not filled out exhaustively. In fact, after checking the tools, only 29% of providers filled them in exhaustively. Filling out the management tools exhaustively makes it possible to monitor and evaluate the system properly, but it also ensures that the receiving facility has all the information it needs to manage the patient.

5.6. THE SYSTEMATIC INCLUSION REFERENCE/COUNTER-REFERENCE BULLETIN AT THE TIME OF REFERENCING

Reference standards require that all references be accompanied by

a reference bulletin/counter reference. The results this study showed that 41

% of referrals made in the Kédougou health district in 2019 were not systematically accompanied by a referral / counter-referral form. Sometimes a handwritten note was written on a blank sheet of paper instead of the referral/counter-referral form.

5.7. THE INCLUSION OF OBSTETRIC EMERGENCY REFERRALS AS AN ITEM ON THE AGENDA OF COORDINATION MEETINGS

Interviews conducted with providers in the Kédougou health district as part of this study revealed that referral of obstetric emergencies is not included as an item on the agenda of coordination meetings. After checking existing coordination meeting reports, referral of obstetric emergencies was never on the agenda.

5.8. EVALUATION OF THE REFERENCE AND CONTROL SYSTEM AGAINST REFERENCE

In 2017, a joint supervision mission by the M.S.A.S with the support of its partners assessed the reference and counter-reference system in the Kédougou region. It was a 5-day supervision mission for the three districts. Given the complexity of the reference and counter-reference system, 5 days would not be enough to evaluate this system. We are not aware of any other evaluation of the reference/counter-reference system up to the time of our study. This shows the weakness of the follow-up evaluation of the reference/counter-reference system.

5.9. SUGGESTIONS FROM SERVICE PROVIDERS FOR IMPROVING THE REFERENCE AND CONTROL SYSTEM AGAINST REFERENCE

The results of the study on the referral and counter-referral system in the Kédougou health district in 2019 revealed several difficulties. Interviews with patients and providers enabled us to highlight the many difficulties faced by referred patients and those involved in the referral and counter-referral system. They made recommendations for improvement. The following graph summarises the various suggestions made by providers during the interviews.

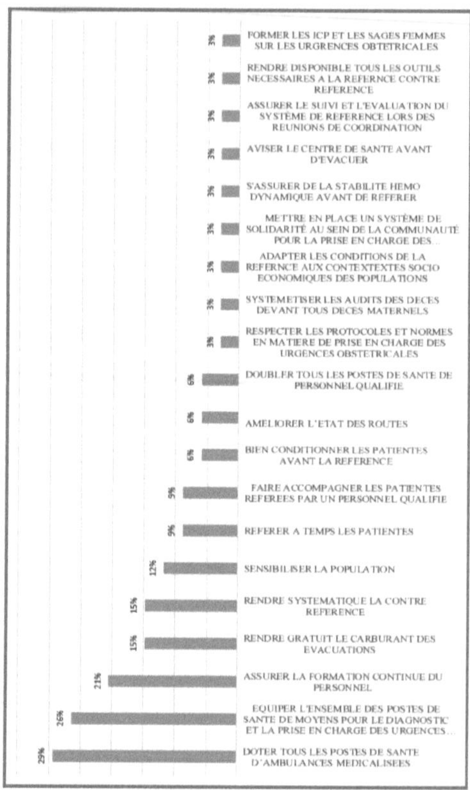

Figure 7: Suggestions from providers.

To this end, 29% of providers suggested that all health facilities should be provided with medical ambulances to enable evacuation under the best possible conditions. The results of this study showed that no facility in the Kédougou health district has a medical ambulance. Instead, simple (non-medicalised) ambulances are available, and these do not guarantee proper management of obstetric emergencies. To resolve the difficulties of the referral and counter-referral system, 26% of providers also suggested making sufficient resources available to service points for the diagnosis and management of obstetric emergencies. As part of improving the referral and counter-referral system, ongoing training for providers is also recommended. To this end, 21% of health workers believe that ongoing training through workshops on basic obstetric and neonatal care (SONUB) would help to improve the referral and counter-referral system. Another solution proposed by the providers is the systematic use of counter-referral (15% of providers). The counter-referral, which is an administrative task aimed at redirecting the patient after her stay in the referral facility with the counter-referral section of the referral bulletin, is not applied at all in the Kédougou health district. All the providers interviewed felt that they had never received a counter-referral, even though this is part of the continuity of the patient's care. Free transport was a frequent solution proposed by providers (15% of providers). In the Kédougou health district, patients pay for fuel when they are evacuated. It is only in cases of extreme emergency that the health development committees pay for fuel for evacuation. The committees are obliged to operate in this way because they do not have a substantial budget to cover the cost of transport for all the patients to be evacuated.

The other solutions recommended by the service providers are as follows:

- Raising public awareness.

- Refer patients in good time.

- Referred patients are accompanied by qualified staff

- Patients should be well conditioned before referral.

- Improving road conditions.

- Double the number of qualified staff in all health posts.

- Comply with protocols and standards for dealing with obstetric emergencies.
- Systematise death audits for all maternal deaths.

- Adapting reference conditions to people's socio-economic backgrounds.
- Set up a community solidarity to cover obstetric referrals.
- Ensure haemodynamic stability before referring.

- Notify the health centre evacuating.

- Monitoring and evaluating the reference system at coordination meetings.
- Make available all the tools needed for reference against reference

- Training ICPs and midwives in obstetric emergencies.

Most of the suggestions made by providers for improving the referral and counter-referral system were related to increasing resources (medical ambulances, equipment for diagnosing and dealing with obstetric emergencies) and building the capacity of Kédougou health district staff. Almost all of the suggestions relate to the 3rd delay (Quality of care received at the referral health facility as soon as possible).

CHAPTER 6

DISCUSSIONS

Our study has enabled us to identify a number of constraints hindering the smooth operation of the reference and counter-reference system.A functional referral and counter-referral system for obstetric emergencies that meets standards can resolve many difficulties. To this end, multi-sectoral approaches are needed to resolve the many constraints linked to the smooth running of the referral and counter-referral system for obstetric emergencies in the Kédougou health district. The health authorities alone cannot resolve these constraints. The health, social action, education and infrastructure sectors, as well as local authorities and communities, need to work together to overcome these constraints. To achieve this, the first step is to avoid the first delay by adopting a good strategy for raising public awareness of obstetric emergencies. As behaviour change is a long process, it is necessary to increase public awareness of obstetric emergencies to avoid the first delay.The results of this study have shown that none of the health facilities in the Kédougou health district have medical ambulances, so there is an urgent need to equip all the facilities with ambulances to ensure continuity of medical and obstetric care during the transfer of patients.The shortage of qualified human resources in the Kédougou health district is an open secret. According to the results of this study, 71% of referrals are not accompanied by qualified staff. The providers interviewed believe that this lack of support is linked to a shortage of qualified human resources. The absence of qualified providers during referral exposes patients to obstetric complications. Therefore, in order to guarantee patient safety during evacuations, it is necessary to reinforce all service points with qualified human resources and double the number of Maternity Units in the health posts in order to make up for the absence of the midwife or the ICP if they are to accompany patients during referral.As part of the drive to improve the referral-to-referral system, the technical facilities at the Maternity Ward of the Kédougou Health Centre need to be improved so that all obstetric emergencies referred can be dealt with effectively.The MSAS has put in place tools for managing the referral and counter-referral system (register/evacuation book, two-part referral and counter-referral form, overall zone report) to provide information. These are good tools that enable all the health information relating to reference and counter-reference activities to be filled in exhaustively. For better monitoring and evaluation of the referral and counter-referral system, all these tools should be available at the service points.The referral and counter-referral system cannot function properly without an effective counter-referral. The counter-referral is a very important step in the management of the patient, as it allows better follow-up of the patient at the peripheral level. The counter-referral must be systematic for all patients referred. It is necessary to designate a person to deal with this administrative task on a full-time basis to facilitate the patient's return to the referring facility. 47% of the patients who took part in this study were dissatisfied with the quality of obstetric emergency care at the Maternity Unit of the Kédougou Health Centre. The population of Kédougou generally deplores the quality of the reception service, although this not been backed up by a scientific study. As reception is part care, providers should improve the quality of reception. Involving communities in the health effort, particularly in the referral and counter-referral system, will help to reduce the constraints linked to the smooth running of this system With a system of community solidarity to cover the cost of evacuation, delays linked to a lack of financial resources could be avoided. Involving the community in the health effort would provide a common understanding of referral and counter-referral issues in order to help the community define its needs and resources in terms of referral and counter-referral and move on to concrete action. As health is a transferred responsibility, local authorities should be involved in the referral and counter-referral system, as health posts alone cannot ensure that the system works properly. Many of the parameters for setting up a good system are beyond their reach. The MSAS authorities should embark on a drive to digitalise the healthcare system, which would enable the reference and counter-reference system to be dematerialised. The referring facility will simply fill in the electronic form and send it to the referring facility, which will in turn make the counter-referral electronically at the end of the patient's hospital stay. This opportunity can be seized to reduce the constraints linked to the smooth running of the referral and counter-referral system by systematising the counter-referral referral forms and improving the monitoring and evaluation of this system.The establishment of a regional consultation framework for the management of the referral and counter-referral system, steered by the medical region, will enable better coordination of referral and counter-referral activities. This will be a framework for planning, monitoring and evaluating referral vs. counter-referral activities, made up of management teams from the medical region and the districts, to improve coordination of the referral vs. counter-referral system.

CONCLUSION

With the aim of providing equitable access to healthcare services for the entire population, and in the context of improving primary healthcare, the referral and counter-referral system has been set up in Senegal to meet the needs of the population in terms of quality of care. The objective of this study was to describe the constraints linked to the smooth running of the referral and counter-referral system for obstetric emergencies at the Maternity Hospital of the Kédougou Health Centre. This description was made through a situational analysis of the referral and counter-referral of obstetric emergencies, then we proceeded to an analysis of the conditions of the referral and counter-referral of obstetric emergencies from the point of view of the providers and from the point of view of the referred patients.

The situational analysis showed that the referral and counter-referral system faces several constraints in the Kédougou health district. None of the facilities has a medical ambulance. Delivery haemorrhage is the main obstetric emergency referred in the Kédougou health district, accounting for 67% of referrals.

The telephone is the most frequently used means of informing the reception structure of the referral decision. However, there is a lack of qualified support for referrals. Lack of human resources obliges providers to have patients accompanied by a matron. Only 29% of patients referred were accompanied by a qualified provider.

All the management tools for the referral and counter-referral system made available to health facilities by the Senegalese Ministry of Health and Social Action (global zone report, two-part referral and counter-referral bulletins and evacuation register/book) are not available in all the health facilities in the Kédougou health district. Furthermore, referral is not systematic after the patient's stay at the maternity ward of the Kédougou health centre. Referral conditions leave much to be desired, according to providers. 76% of the health workers surveyed considered referral conditions for obstetric emergencies to be "very difficult" because of "the lack of practicable roads", "the lack of qualified human resources", etc. to accompany patients when they are evacuated, "transport is not free", "patients are poorly conditioned when they arrive" and "there are no medical ambulances". In the Kédougou health district, none of the facilities has a medical ambulance. Instead of medical ambulances, simple ambulances are used for evacuations, and these do not guarantee compliance with patient transport standards and procedures. On the whole, the patients referred appreciated the referral conditions, but some patients were not satisfied because of the length of time between their arrival at the facility and their treatment, and the absence of a reception and referral service at the Maternity Ward of the Kédougou Health Centre. The results of this study also showed a weakness in the monitoring and documentation of the reference and counter-reference system. Not all the management tools are filled in exhaustively. A referral and counter-referral bulletin is not issued systematically at the time of referral, and after checking existing coordination meeting reports, referral of obstetric emergencies is never on the agenda. Apart from the joint MSAS supervision mission carried out in 2017, no other evaluation of the referral and counter-referral system has been brought to our attention up to the time of our study. We can therefore answer in the affirmative in relation to our research hypothesis and say that the poor performance of the referral and counter-referral system is linked to the weakness of the monitoring and documentation of referral and counter-referral. The Kédougou Health District does not have a monitoring and evaluation plan for the following indicators: reasons for referral, accompaniment by a qualified service provider during referral, means of transport used during referral, use of a referral and counter-referral form, compliance with counter-referral by patients. No system can be effective without regular monitoring and evaluation. Monitoring and documentation make it possible to evaluate the reference and counter-reference system, rectify anomalies in the system and correct them in order to have a high-performance reference and counter-reference system capable of meeting the needs of providers and patients.

REFERENCES BIBLIOGRAPHIQUES

1. Baldé, I. S., et al. (2019). Determinants of obstetrical complications on the arrival of parturients at Conakry University Hospital in relation to 645 observations. Determinants of Obstetrical. Rev int sc méd Abj -RISM-2019;21,3:175-179.

2. Boré, B. (2021). Evaluation du système de référence-évacuation des urgences obstétricales du district sanitaire de Macina de 2017à 2019 (Doctoral dissertation, USTTB).

3. Dembélé, H. (2020). Evaluation du système de référence/évacuation axe sur les urgences obstétricales de 2015 à 2018 dans le District Sanitaire de Yelimané (Doctoral dissertation, Université des Sciences, des Techniques et des Technologies de Bamako), 92 pages.

4. Diallo, A., et al. (2019). Evaluation of the reference and counter-reference system obstetrical care at Ignace Deen maternity hospital in Guinea. Jaccr Africa, 3(4), 505-516.

5. Houngnihin, R. A., & Sossou, A. J. (2017). Understanding obstetric referral renunciation at the Cotonou University Clinic Gynecology and Obstetrics. Santé Publique, 29(5), 719-729.

6. Kafuku, M. (2016). L'analyse comparative opérationnelle de la référence et contre référence en milieu urbain et rural: cas des Zones de Santé Kisanga et Kapolowe, University of Lubumbashi, 67 pages.

7. N'golo, F. (2018). Evaluation of the referral/evacuation system for obstetric emergencies at the CS ref CIV in the district of Bamako. Thesis in medicine. Université des sciences des techniques et des technologies de Bamako, 107 pages.

8. Ngom, N. F. (2016). L'assistance médicale à l'accouchement au Sénégal (Doctoral dissertation, University of Bordeaux).

9. Pires, A. (1997). Échantillonnage et recherche qualitative: essai théorique et méthodologique. La recherche qualitative. Enjeux épistémologiques et méthodologiques, 64-68.

10. Tchaou, B. A., et al. (2015). Obstetric emergencies at Parakou University Hospital in Benin: clinical, therapeutic and evolutionary aspects. European Scientific Journal, 11(9).

11. Théra, T., et al. (2015). Problematique du système de référence-contre-référence des urgences obstétricales et l'implication des communautés dans le district de Bamako. Mali médical, 30(3).

12. Thiam, M. (2017). Maternal mortality at the Centre Hospitalier Régional de Thiès: aetiologies and determining factors, about 239 deaths. JOURNAL OF SAGO (Gynaecology-

Obstetrics and Reproductive Health), 18(1).

13. Thiam, O. (2014). La problématique des parturientes évacuées en zone rurale sénégalaise: exemple du centre hospitalier de Ndioum. Revue Africaine et Malgache de Recherche Scientifique/Sciences de la Santé, 1(2).

14. Touré, S. (2019). Evaluation of the obstetric referral/evacuation system at the Banamba referral health centre. Thesis in Medicine. University of sciences of techniques and technologies of Bamako, 91 pages.

15. Traoré, A. T. (2014). Obstetrical emergencies in the context of referral evacuation at the Major Moussa Diakité referral health centre in Kati à propos de 319 cases. Université des sciences des techniques et des technologies de Bamako, 87 pages.

16. Traoré, D. (2010). Problématique du système de référence/évacuation des urgences obstétricales au CS de référence du district sanitaire de Bamako (Doctoral dissertation, Thèse de Méd. Bamako), 130 pages.

17. Vancutsem, I. (2011). Analysis of the reference and counter reference system in the savannah region of northern Togo. Internship report. 52 pages.

18. World Health Organization. (2015). Tracking universal health coverage: first global monitoring report. World Health Organization.

WEBOGRAPHY

1. https://senegal.dhis2.org/ visited on 24 September 2020.

2. https://www.ansd.sn/ressources/publications/Rapport-final-EHCVM-vf-Senegal.pdf visited on 07 February 2022.

3. https://www.sec.gouv.sn/publications/lois-et-reglements/loi-ndeg-2001-03-du-22- january-2001-bearing-constitution-amended. Visited on 19 March 2020.

4. https://www.ansd.sn/ressources/rapports/Rapport%20Final%20EDS%202017.pdf visited on 09 April 2020.

5. https://www.gieraf.org/assets/images/article_41/01SONU%20AFRIQUE%203%C3% A8me%20%C3%A9dition%202018.pdf visited on 05 August 2022.

APPENDICES

APPENDIX 1: QUESTIONNAIRE FOR QUALIFIED HEALTHCARE STAFF

STUDY ON THE CONSTRAINTS LINKED TO THE SMOOTH RUNNING OF THE REFERRAL AND COUNTER-REFERRAL SYSTEM FOR OBSTETRIC EMERGENCIES AT THE KEDOUGOU HEALTH CENTRE MATERNITY HOSPITAL IN 2019 BY MAMADOU MOUSTAPHA THIOUB

Questionnaire on the constraints linked to the smooth running of the referral and counter-referral system for obstetric emergencies at the Maternity Hospital of the Kédougou Health Centre in 2019.

IDENTIFICATION OF THE HEALTH FACILITY MEDICAL REGION OF KEDOUGOU HEALTH DISTRICT OF KEDOUGOU TYPE OF STRUCTURE :

MAINTENANCE INFORMATION		
DATE OF INTERVIEW		
START TIME	END TIME	
A) SITUATIONAL ANALYSIS OF REFERENCE/COUNTER-REFERENCE ACTIVITIES		
1. HEALTH POST LEVEL		
No.	QUESTIONS	ANSWERS NB: for closed questions, put (1) for YES or (2) for NO
1	To which of the following types of facilities do you usually refer your obstetric emergencies? (s) answer(s)) :	
	-Health post	| |
	-Health centre	| |
	-EPS	| |
	-Private practice/clinic	| |
2	THE REFERENCE	

	Does the head of post or the midwife use the algorithms in the MSAS policies, protocols and standards for managing obstetric emergencies?	1|	|2|	|	
	He/she decides on the reference by ensuring that:				
	-The patient is well stabilised before transport (emergency medicines available)	1|	|2|	|	
	-The family has received all the information on the terms of reference	1|	|2|	|	
3	-He/she ensures that the transport is carried out promptly, safely and promptly	1|	|2|	|	
4	All forms are completed full before departure: Consultation register, Register/reference book Reference sheet ?	1.|	|	|	|
	Do you inform the host organisation that a patient referred?	1.|	|	|	|
	If so, how? (Tick right answer(s)) :	|	|		
	-A standard reference form (with reference and counter-reference flaps)	|	|		
	-A handwritten note	|	|		
5	-Telephone	|	|		
	-Support by a service provider qualified	|	|		
	-Other (please specify)	|	|		
	If not, why not?				
6	Are the concerns of the patient or those accompanying her regularly taken into account in terms of facilities, cost, transport and hours?	1.|	|	|	|
7	When do you inform the receiving facility of the decision to refer your patient? (Tick the right answer(s)) :				
	Before the patient left?	|	|		
	When the patient leaves?	|	|		

	After the patient has left?	|	|			
8	Who decided on the reference? (Tick the right answer(s)) :					
	-Community health actors (ACS)	|	|			
	-Head nurse (ICP)	|	|			
	-Master midwife/Midwife	|	|			
	-The patient or her family	|	|			
	-Other (please specify)	|	|			
9	Does the structure have a means of transport for references?	1.|	|	|	|	
	If YES, which ones? (Tick the right box(es))(s) answer(s)) :					
	- Bicycle/motorcycle	|	|			
	- Vehicle	|	|			
	- Public transport	|	|			
	- Tricycle ambulance	|	|			
	- Simple ambulance	|	|			
	- Medical ambulance	|	|			
	- Other: please specify					
10	If a medical ambulance is used, are the following items available inside the vehicle in the event of evacuation? (Tick the right box(es))(s) answer(s)) :					
	-Resuscitation equipment: oxygen, defibrillator, emergency kit (batch of medicines and consumables	|	|			
	-Functional equipment for one track	|	|			
	venous					
	-Qualified accompanying staff	|	|			
11	Does your organisation have the following management tools? (check the different tools)					
	-Reference/counter-reference bulletin in two parts	1.|	|	|	|	
	-Monthly report on the activities of the reference and counter-reference	1.|	|	|	|	
	-Evacuation register/book.	1.|	|	|	|	

		THE COUNTER REFERENCE				
12	The head of the referral department confirms or gives instructions the ICP or midwife on the reason for the referral and gives indications for follow-up?	1.|	|	2|	|
13	Has your organisation been informed that a patient was counter-referred?	1.|	|	2|	|
14	If so, by what means? (Tick correct answer(s) :				
	-A counter reference form standard	|	|		
	-A handwritten note	|	|		
	-A telephone call	|	|		
B) Referral and counter-referral conditions for obstetric emergencies in the provider's point of view.						
15	Which are the main obstetric emergencies referred by your facility (Health post level)				
16	What are the main obstetric emergencies referred to your facility? (Maternity level)				
17	qualified personnel available? Enough supplies 24 hours a day to deal with obstetric emergencies?	1.|	|	|	|
18	Is que the standards in for reference standards are met before the departure of the patient?	1.	|	|	2|
19	Is referral to qualified staff systematic for all emergencies? obstetrics?	1.	|	|	2|
20	Do you have a medical ambulance?for obstetric emergencies?	1.	|	|	2|
21	Are all evacuated patients properly conditioned on arrival at maternity hospital?The Kédougou health centre?	1.	|	|	2|
22	Does your organisation have sufficient resources for the care in care of obstetric emergencies?	1.	|	|	2|
23	What suggestions do you have for improving the reference and counter-reference system? Referral of obstetric emergencies?	1.	|	|	2|

No.	QUESTIONS	ANSWERS
24	How would you rate the referral conditions obstetric emergencies in your facility? (Describe your answer)	
C) THE DELAY IN THE REFERENCE'S DECISION-MAKING PROCESS		
No.	QUESTIONS	ANSWERS
23	Are service providers trained in emergency protocols?	1.| | | |
24	Is there a long delay (more than 30 minutes) between the patient's arrival and the referral decision? (Check exhaust register)	1.| | | |
25	Between patients evacuated on time and patients evacuated with a delay in the decision, which have a higher success rate?	Set (1) for patients evacuated on time or (2) for patients evacuated with a delay in decision-making 1. | | | |
26	Are the maternal deaths recorded in your facility very often linked to the delay in taking the decision to evacuate?	1.| | | |
27	Do you think that the delay in deciding on the reference may be an obstacle to the proper functioning of the reference and counter-reference system?	1.| | | |
D) WEAK MONITORING AND DOCUMENTATION OF THE REFERENCE AND COUNTER-REFERENCE		
28	Do you have an evacuation and reference / counter reference bulletins? (Check existence of the register and the bulletins if yes)	1.| | | |
29	Are all the items in the register and on the forms completed in full?	1.| | | |
30	Are references accompanied by systematically a reference bulletin /against reference?	1.| | | |
31	Is the referral of obstetric emergencies included as an item on the agenda of coordination meetings? (Check coordination meeting report)	1.| | | |
	Is information on referrals for obstetric emergencies taken into account in activity reports? ?	1.| | | |
32	Has the reference and counter-reference system already been evaluated?	1.| | | |

APPENDIX 2: INTERVIEW GUIDE FOR PREGNANT WOMEN IN LABOUR OR POST PARTUM.

STUDY ON THE CONSTRAINTS LINKED TO THE SMOOTH RUNNING OF THE REFERRAL AND COUNTER-REFERRAL SYSTEM FOR OBSTETRIC EMERGENCIES AT THE KEDOUGOU HEALTH CENTRE MATERNITY HOSPITAL IN 2019 BY MAMADOU MOUSTAPHA THIOUB.

Interview guide on the constraints linked to the smooth running of the referral and counter-referral system for obstetric emergencies at the Maternity Hospital of the Kédougou Health Centre in 2019.

MAINTENANCE INFORMATION			
DATE OF INTERVIEW			
START TIME		END TIME	
Referral and counter-referral conditions for obstetric emergencies in the the point of view of the evacuees/accompanying persons.			
No.	QUESTIONS	ANSWERS NB: for closed questions, put (1) for YES or (2) for NO	
1	Are the reasons for the referral always explained to you after the appointment? decision to evacuate?	1. |	2| |
2	At of your evacuation, were you accompanied by a qualified health worker?	1. |	2| |
3	Have you received any pre-transfer treatment before your evacuation?	1. | |	2| |
4	What means of transport did you use?		
5	Were the evacuation costs free?	1. | |	2| |
6	How do you rate the time between your arrival in the department and the taking of your appointment? decision to evacuate you?		
7	Is there a system of solidarity within the community for the provision of care? obstetrical references?	1. | |	2| |
8	Have you received a counter reference to the end of your hospital stay?	1. | |	2| |
9	How do you assess the quality of obstetric emergencies?		
10	How do you rate the conditions under which obstetric emergencies are referred to the hospital? (Describe your answer)		

APPENDIX 3: REFERENCE SHEET AGAINST REFERENCE

REFERENCE/COUNTER-REFERENCE SHEET

Structure

ORIGIN :
OF DESTINATION :

Name of health worker:

Position:

Name of person referred:

Age:

Years/Months

Sex M/F Precise address:

CPC NUMBER:

Arrived at the facility on at hour(s)minute(s)

Time of

Decision-making :

Leaving the structure :

Physiological constants: BP ..Pulse: ./mn T°c..Weight kg FR../mn

Reason of the reference :

Date

AGAINST REFERENCE

Patient's name: .

Age:

Years/Months

Sex M/F Precise address :

N° in the consultation register :

Referred by

Arrived on at .h.mn

Reason of the reference :

Viewed on:at H..mn By

Function

Diagnosis

Entrance :

Out :

Treatment

RECOMMENDATIONS FOR MONITORING AT STRUCTURE LEVEL

ORIGIN

Date

Signature and stamp

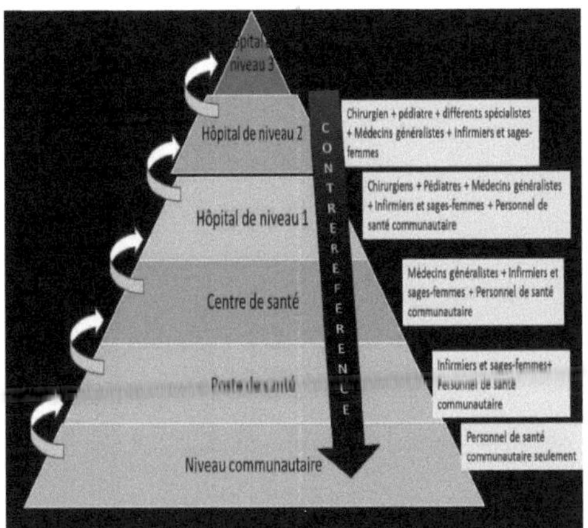

Hôpital niveau 3
Hôpital de niveau 2
Hôpital de niveau 1
Centre de santé
Poste de santé
Niveau communautaire
CONTRE REFERENCE
Chirurgien + pédiatre + différents spécialistes + Médecins généralistes + Infirmiers et sages-femmes
Chirurgiens + Pédiatres + Médecins généralistes + Infirmiers et sages-femmes + Personnel de santé communautaire
Médecins généralistes + Infirmiers et sages-femmes + Personnel de santé communautaire
Infirmiers et sages-femmes+ Personnel de santé communautaire
Personnel de santé communautaire seulement

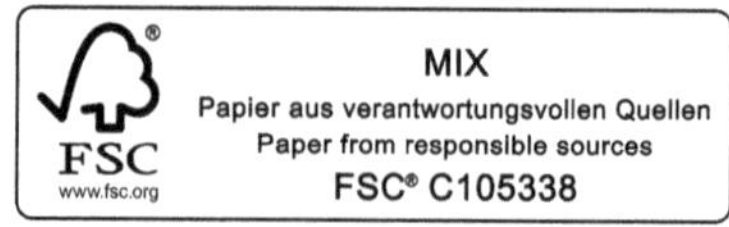

Printed by Books on Demand GmbH, Norderstedt / Germany